Medical Billing and Coding Beginners Guide

Comprehensive Medical Coding & Billing Book

Millie Reddington

Contents

Introduction

The aspect or system of medical billing and coding has been one important part of the health care structure. Its place secures a sense of control on major areas dealing with finance and has been described as the "heart" of the medical industry.

A look into coding and billing processes isn't all centered on different kinds of codes or jargon given out by someone having specialized knowledge about an organization. It basically has to do with creating an existing working relationship between individuals and businesses, in this case, patients and health care professionals, down to other coders and representatives of insurance.

One main purpose of our visit to the hospital is to see improvement in our well-being. All we do is check in on the date of our appointment, make consultations, supply all necessary information about our medical insurer, then make a payment, also known as a copay. Copay is just part of the total amount to be paid for a visit to the hospital. It's possible we haven't given it a thought on how the healthcare system is being run, that is, how its financial system is being handled. Of course, the health care workers, the hospital itself, and other factors, which are very effective in running the health industry, need some form of payment for services rendered. The copay is not just the payment made. There are some others that cover a major portion of the cost (of service). That is where the medical insurer comes in. The insurer makes payment of the total cost. This is done after the necessary submission of an insurance claim by the health worker, coupled with other documents, which can serve as a form of backup or proof that a service was indeed rendered on a visit. This claim is well scrutinized and approved, with corresponding pay given to the health worker.

Over time, this billing system has maintained a record of efficiency in processes relating to expenses in the medical field, observed especially from concerned patients. A health worker provides all manner of care spanning different types of treatments and medical procedures to a large number of patients on a daily basis. This is definitely a daunting task even though such personnel have been adequately trained. Then, try to picture a situation where such a person is required to provide documents, bills, or other paperwork, for each patient seen and treated daily and do the same for the next day. This can be very tasking indeed. Any errors made during this process can lead to a delay in payment. Financial crisis becomes the other of the day as the health personnel plunges deeply, as a result of irregular or depleted means of payment from insurers. The reason isn't far-fetched. Apart from errors that can lead to delay in payment, huge forms of expenses can be made by a health worker. This is normal for the proper running of the industry. A health worker in charge needs to provide for medical and administrative welfare, make payments for hospital supplies, rent, and other utilities, to provide the best form of care to patients. It then becomes a problem when the reimbursement fails to actualize after expenses have been made.

Several issues have been found to have a huge impact on payment made by a medical insurer to the health worker. It is possible that the insurer rebuts claims made or causes a form of delay in processing the payment. This mostly occurs because of errors in billing and coding. Another can be avoidable or unavoidable errors, and it is until the health worker is able to lay appropriate claims that the situation can be resolved.

The scale of financial constraints can become out-weighing on a health care worker and can only be relieved by insurance payment. He or she is, up to a certain extent, bestowed with the ability to offer quality care to patients and see to their well-being, not trying to wrap their heads on issues surrounding billing and coding or insurance policies, rules, and regulations. This is why the importance of medical insurers or insurance specialists cannot be overemphasized.

Medical insurance specialists are experts on medical billing and coding and can be relied upon by health care providers. These professionals are saddled with the tasks of preparing claims and the necessary paper works or documents needed for payment or reimbursement to be issued. As a medical insurance specialist, it is important you have a good grasp on procedures pertaining to the medical office, be skilled in procedure coding, understand how medical insurance plans work, resolve any dispute which arises on claims, have the required ability to make use of medical management software, and more skills. Just a glance at these gives off the feeling of complexity. Well, that's no surprise, but it shouldn't put you off. The skills are learnable as they have maintained a track record of offering impeccable solutions to tasks that seem impossible to solve, used by insurance specialists daily. Medical billing and coding explore these techniques, and you can get to apply them in daily clinical practice, putting away any form of apprehension, delay, or indecision in attaining this specialty.

Chapter 1: What Is Medical Billing And Coding?

The terrain of medical billing and coding is open to all as it has a greater impact on the lives of every individual in the health care sector than some other jobs in that field. These individuals are seen as important as their welfare tells a story to the outside world about the medical sector.

The amount of individuals seeking to offer their services in the healthcare sector is on the rise. The industry is booming, no doubt, whether one is directly involved in taking care of patients or working somewhere else, within.

A statistical analysis by the Bureau of Labor Statistics has projected a significant rise in the industry centering on medical billing and coding. The value projected is a 22% increase, coursing through 2026. This clearly shows that it is a very robust market for investment. That's one smart move and a good time to take part.

One very common notion about the medical industry is that doctors and nurses take up a major part in effectively running the system. They are majorly seen to be actively involved in taking care of patients in the hospital. Well, that observation is true from a perspective, but not entirely. There are underground personalities making sure that things around the hospitals or other medical facilities work. They see the possibility of bridging the gap between the patients and the health care worker. Some good examples involved are medical billing and coding processes. Running an administration with the skills of billing and coding improves functionality within the healthcare system.

The field of medical billing and coding is on an advancing level in the healthcare sector and has proven to be quite important. Applying medical billing and coding to modern health care practices are closely related, although in an actual sense, separate entities. They work hand in hand to achieve a goal of ensuring necessary payments for health care services rendered; that is, the reimbursement cycle is very active and well streamlined.

You can see professionals or specialists of medical billing and coding in different facility types ranging from hospitals, medical offices, centers for rehabilitation, and other departments of health. Work activities are usually carried out in an environment likened to an office. A specialist in medical billing and coding can work on a full-time basis or part-time due to the organization of the medical facility. In terms of dressing, they can put on clothing as directed by the employer or suitable for the setting. In some other settings, scrubs are worn the same as that of the clinical staff.

The two skills are described individually, below.

Medical Billing

Medical billing is one very essential process that sees to the proper and smooth functioning of a medical facility or hospital. In this case, billing claims are created and delivered to the insurance providers. On final assessment, it is ensured that the hospital or medical facility is being paid the amount proportional to the care, treatment, or services rendered to the patients.

Funding of the hospital body or medical facility can come from different sources. One of such is from private insurance providers and another, healthcare programs, which have been arraigned by the government. Funding is necessary. A good amount of funds will go a long way in keeping the healthcare system in the business line. Reimbursements, which are below par, will pose a lot of problems for medical facilities as they will find it difficult to offer quality services to patients.

To understand the concept of medical billing, let's take a look at a patient coming down with a productive cough (a cough that is not dry and with lots of mucus production) and feeling feverish. Such a patient books an appointment with the doctor, signaling the start of the medical billing process. The nurse quizzes the patient on various symptoms being experienced and has some tests carried out at the initial stages. This is followed by an examination done by the doctor and then, a diagnosis, in this case, bronchitis. The appropriate medications are then prescribed.

The already prepared codes are gotten by the biller. Such codes are indications for the disease condition and symptoms experienced by the patient, the type of visit, what has been diagnosed by the doctor, and the prescriptions made. After code preparation, the biller creates claims from them using a special kind of software. These claims are then sent to the insurance company, and on working on it, sends it back to the biller. The biller also performs their own evaluation of the returned claim. Here, an assessment is made on the total amount to be paid by the patient, and a deduction of the amount of insurance has been made.

The patient showcasing these symptoms, characteristics of bronchitis, will pay a relatively low amount on the condition of having an insurance cover over the visit to the doctor and subsequent treatment(s) provided. A part-payment known as copay can be made by the patient or possibly, come to an agreement with the insurance company offering them such services. The biller then processes all these and forms the correct bill. It is ensured that the bill gets to the hands of the patient.

Some situations can arise where patients decline payment of bills. In such cases, the medical biller has the responsibility of seeking the services of a collection agency. An agency such as these sees to the proper compensation of the healthcare provider.

You can conclude that the medical biller acts as a link between the patient, health care worker, and that of the insurance company. See the biller as a translator performing the act of transforming codes into reports covering financial analysis. The biller has quite a lot of responsibilities, but such can be rounded up to ensure proper reimbursement of the healthcare worker for the quality of services rendered.

Medical Coding

Medical coding, as the case may be, is also an important aspect of making insurance reimbursement. It specifically has to do with assigning special codes for every form of care or service provided, ranging from diagnosis to that of assigned treatments and prescriptions. These diagnoses, treatments or procedures, and prescriptions are transformed into universal codes, thereby according to the health care worker the means to process the bill in the correct manner.

Medical coding grew out of the reason to keep things precise and short so that they can be well handled. The method of coding medically has to do with transforming the medical diagnosis, treatments, and also, equipment into numeric or alphanumeric medical codes. These codes are built into a form of combination. The coder does the work of taking what is written by the medical officer; the diagnosis, treatments, and prescription for a medication, and gets it translated. Doing this makes it easy for documents to be uniform, well-structured and go a long way in making it easier for the administration to identify how effective treatment works and the prevalence. The codes are specific for every visit by the patient, symptoms exhibited, diagnoses, and procedures, and there's always a code in correspondence.

Taking a look at the case study of bronchitis used earlier, there is an accorded recording of every action carried out by the patient during the visit, done by either the doctor or someone within the office of the health worker. The medical coder's job is to get every bit of information about the patient's visit translated into numeric and alphanumeric codes, which is needed for the billing process.

Different sets and subsets of codes exist, and as a medical coder, you must be well associated with them. Two common codes which exist are: International Classification of Diseases (ICD) codes and Current Procedure Terminology (CPT). The ICD focuses on conditions of injuries or illnesses associated with a patient, while that of the CPT deals with professional services meted out by the healthcare worker for the patient. The codes used are well known by every doctor, hospital, government agency, insurance company and clearinghouse, and other forms of organization associated with health.

As there are different sets of codes, so also is the availability of their guidelines and rules. Some codes need to be arranged in a particular order especially that of the ones showing a pre-existing condition. It is important that every code should be done accurately and follow the appropriate guidelines as it can affect the claim status.

At the final stages, the medical coder inputs the necessary codes in the appropriate forms or software. Once coding is completed, the report is then sent to the medical biller.

Types of Coding

Current Procedural Terminology (CPT)

This type of coding has to do with the different forms of services provided by health care professionals, which includes surgical operations, tests, and others. The maintenance of this set of codes is by the American Medical Association (AMA). The AMA carries out regular renewal of these codes to showcase the necessary changes in the medical field. Three classes of CPT codes exist:

Category 1: Codes pertaining to the procedures and services, well described. They are five in number.

Category 2: These are alphanumeric codes for tracking and are suitable for measuring executions.

Category 3: These are the provisional codes suitable for services, technologies, and procedures that are just coming up.

International Classification of Diseases (ICD)

The World Health Organization (WHO) refers to ICD as the standard by which diseases and other health conditions are defined, internationally. In this case, the set codes are applied in identifying the trending health concerns and the available statistics. The latest edition of ICD is that of the 10th edition, and there have been several updates on the editions, done by health workers and payers. A proposed 11th edition is on the way, prepared to be implemented in January 2022.

The ICD, edition 10, together with all its components, also a product of the World Health Organization, are quite important for processes that have to do with billing and recording, and also for keeping accurate records of information on diseases, nationally and worldwide.

Healthcare Common Procedure Coding (HCPCS)

This coding focuses on two levels of code set that deals majorly with medical equipment, ambulance services, prosthetics, care for outpatients, supplies, chemothera-py drugs, and others. These codes don't relate directly in any way to the health worker. Changes are made to the set, which depends on the feedback given by the public.

International Classification of Functioning, Disability, and Health (ICF)

This has dealings with the structure of the body and its functions, disabilities, how patient's activities and active participation are impacted, information centering on the severity and factors present in the environment.

Diagnosis Related Groups (DRG)

DRG is based more on Medicare patients. Every form of information and condition of these patients are arranged in categories. Due to the fact that a previous classification of the categories has been made, there's an assumption by Medicare that the patient needs the same form of care and proceeds to issue out a reimbursement, determined by that same level of care.

Medical coding is one important process that a hospital setting can't do without. The type of practice therein will ascertain the kind of medical code set and the coder that will be applied consistently.

Different hospital settings have their own methods of application. For clinics of smaller size, they have different options for activities pertaining to billing and coding. They may take up the use of special software for data entry or use the services of a consultant as a form of outsourcing for coding requirements. That of hospitals with larger organization systems have a department dedicated specifically for coding activities. They can also outsource the activity due to the numerous billboard patients.

Why Should We Code?

You may wonder why medical reports should be coded. Shouldn't we go about listing the symptoms, diagnoses, and procedures of treatment, and then have them sent to the insurance company for processing, to get feed-back on the services due for reimbursement?

Well, there's an estimate by the Centers for Disease Control (CDC) that about 1.4 billion patients visited health care settings. These settings included; outpatient facilities, emergency departments, doctor offices. If an estimate is given on five different coded information on each visit, that is, a very much low estimate, it will produce a total of 6 billion classified pieces of infor-mation that are needed total be transferred each year. A system that deals with a large flow of data needs medical coding to enable the effective transfer of huge bulk of information.

With coding, useful information is well documented in a uniform manner, between facilities. Uniformity is key. A code for streptococcal sore throat can be identified the same way in two different countries. Uniformity of data promotes efficiency in analysis and research activities, and with this, the government and other health agencies can effectively track down various trends in health. For example, if the CDC wants to ascertain the prevalence of pneumonia, they can easily do searches for recent cases of pneumonia diagnoses just by searching for the ICD 10 code.

Finally, an administration can have an overview of how their facility is faring based on the effectiveness of treatment and incidence. A large medical facility like that of tertiary care hospitals needs the services of medical coding companies. The rise in the incidence of a particular disease is tracked by government agencies, so also is the need for medical facilities to track the effectiveness of their services.

Is Medical Billing Different from Medical Coding?

There's a great assumption that billing and coding is just one job function. They are entirely two different careers.

Some differences exist between medical billing and coding. Medical coding kick starts the process of billing and coding, and it involves the application of the appropriate codes to health records and claims. That of medical billing, the second part, involves the transferring of claims to the right quarters; the patients and insurance companies. They cover the necessary costs of treatment or services rendered.

Each job has specific tasks and functions.

The medical coder processes every document that has to do with a patient's visit and interaction with health care workers, such as doctors, nurses, surgeons, and others, and applies the required codes for the procedure (CPT) and diagnosis (ICD), showcasing the services rendered.

The medical biller takes over the codes already assigned and that of other necessary insurance information. These details are inputted into the software designed for billing. The payer, which is usually the insurance company, receives the claim from the medical biller. A form of follow-up is needed on the claim by the medical biller.

Medical billers and coders also perform various tasks and also engage in a regular form of communication with people. These tasks exist:

The reason for billing insurance companies and also patients accords medical billers the necessary form of interaction between them and the patients or insurance companies, to ensure the smooth payment of claims in due time. Well, it isn't such an easy task as patients can get worried or unhappy about the number of bills to be paid or when they get rejected by health insurance companies. Empathy and a great deal of patience are therefore an important need for the medical biller.

For coders, they don't have any interaction with the patients while carrying out their duties. They only deal with records and inputting data. These differences saw the need for different personalities to take up the roles. Introverted and extroverted types of personalities are ideal for different roles. The job of medical billers involves constant communication with insurance companies and patients, tending themselves to the extroverted personality. An introverted personality is ideal for the medical coders as they are, most of the time, working with their computers and records. Sometimes, work involves other healthcare workers, but at most, tasks are mostly independent.

For more accurate coding activities, the medical coder can question the healthcare providers on any issues centering on the procedures or services rendered on patient's visit and also, provide the necessary education on the importance of assembling the right information.

Medical billers also give explanations to patients on the accumulated charges, especially when the patient is finding it difficult to understand what payments are to be made, for example, copayments and coinsurance, specified by the insurance company.

On submission of claims to the insurance company, it is the duty of the medical biller to ascertain that the format of the billing is correct, apply the correct modifiers, and make sure that all necessary documents are submitted with each claim. Both the medical billers and coders are well involved in collecting the necessary information and documents, and also code claims correctly to make sure health care providers are paid in due time. They also ensure proper follow- up of all payers to make sure every payment gets to the health care provider. The functioning of these two jobs is essential in the cash flow system of a healthcare provider, and the running can be done by two different individuals or one person, depending on how big the office is.

There are some certain professional courses that can be done to get one well qualified for a job role. A medical coder can pick from:

Certified Professional Coder (CPC) Certified Coding Associate (CCA) Certified Coding Specialist (CSS)

For medical billers, there's no need to get any professional certification to embark on the role, but it can help in salary negotiation and eventually getting that desired job. The Certified Professional Biller certificate should be something worth considering.

Most billers and coders take part in vocational training programs at colleges. On graduation, they get a certificate of completion. The duration of these programs is usually 1-2 years, and what is usually taught to medical coders and billers, aspiring ones especially, are special types of information dealing with health insurance and terms in the medical field for the smooth running of the job.

Is Medical Billing and Coding a Difficult Field of Healthcare to Get into?

Medical billing and coding are career prospects; therefore, as with other careers, there's a need for one to put in the required interest, dedication and seek out the right information and preparation. There's a need to equip yourself with the skills to go through various code sets and systems of classification, and also, how to go about using software for effective management of patients records, submitting insurance claims, and dealing with billing processes in order to suit the needs of medical billing and coding roles.

One thing with these job roles especially that of medical coding, is that you don't have to memorize all the different codes from the code sets. There are available programs or software that will provide the necessary information on using or applying codebooks and help perform billing and coding processes in an orderly manner.

Importance of Medical Billing and Coding

Applying medical billing and coding in a healthcare facility improves overall productivity. Patients being cared for will be charged the appropriate amount for services rendered and not more. An example is a case where a code is not properly entered, indicating that a particular treatment given to a patient is more expensive than actualized.

Chapter 2: Medical Accounting And Job Coding Prospects

B eing on the lookout for a promising career exposes you to many options. For example, if you're very good with numbers, the option of being an accountant is there, so also is tending towards a role as a healthcare provider, if you have the much-needed feel to spend time seeing to the well-being of people, both physically and mentally. Well, have you considered the option of doing both? What if you've thought of the idea of applying your skills using numbers and making various contributions to a system whose goal is to see people get help? Medical accounting may suit your taste in career choice.

A look from the aspect of finance shows that the healthcare system is quite complex. Different policies and legislation spring up as the market grows, expensive and well-advanced technologies are on the rise, and patients demand more financial transparency. All these will see the need to acquire the services of an accounting professional.

The goal of the healthcare system is to see that individuals (patients) get relief from sicknesses, diseases, and injuries, prevent such, and seek a prolonged healthier life. For medical facilities to run efficiently, there's a need for a budget to be created and rightly followed. A reasonable budget proves effective monitoring of money being spent or money coming into the organization. With this, the facility will have enough cash to carry out its activities. Such a facility won't find it difficult to pay its staff, get supplies, provide care for patients, and more.

Medical accounting professionals carry out the function of gathering, creating analysis, and interpreting financial data. They also keep financial records, balance sheets, cash flow analyses, and other records for hospitals and insurance companies, rendering health-care services. These records give the organization an overview to make relevant decisions.

There exist specific tax rules and auditing necessities, which every health care system must duly follow. These rules can be difficult in terms of their structures and complexities. So, as a thriving health care system, it is necessary to assign a professional with advanced knowledge and skills to navigate the terrains of the rules. These professionals, well trained in medical ac-counting, are very good at handling such tasks. The organization or system will then find it easier to make confident decisions that will benefit all, including all dai-ly activities. Sometimes, the decisions made will have a lingering effect on future planning and programs.

A medical accountant is, in a way, serving the interest of the people, making such a role an essential aspect of the healthcare system.

Value of the Medical Accounting Role

At one point or the other, creating budgets have be-come an intricate part of our lives, but to make one, taking note of the amount of income coming in and accrued bills or expenses, is vital. Also, and at any time, unexpected situations can come up, like a child coming down with sickness, need for a new car, or an accident. Well, how easy is it to manage such occurrences, especially when there's no adequate preparation for such events? It can be a stressful disaster for some.

The above situation can be the same problem with the healthcare system. This is the more reason there's a need for an individual to effectively monitor the inflow and outflow of monies of an organization, thus properly keeping such an organization in business and leading to good rendering of service to people in need.

Medical Accounting and General Accounting. How is it different?

One notable difference between medical accounting and accounting, in general, is that a medical accountant has easy access to vital details or information about a patient. Such details are private, as confidentiality is a watchword in the medical field. The details can be about the disease being suffered from and the type of care provided. Access to these will require concrete adherence to the HIPAA (Health Insurance Portability and Accountability Act) regulations.

The HIPAA seeks to regulate these two practices; good healthcare coverage for people between jobs and proper confidentiality of patients' information.

There's a great probability of patients' details, such as diagnoses, treatments, and medical histories, getting leaked or shared by staff. A good confidentiality system hampers such happenings, even during the process of transferring such vital details to other agencies such as healthcare specialists and professionals, pharmacies, and insurance companies.

With this, it is highly needed that medical accountants collaborate with the HIPAA regulatory system when taking part in roles involving billing and claims submission. These documents usually contain a great deal of information that ought to be confidential.

Accountants in the medical field do work quite similar to that of Certified Public Accountants (CPAs) and other professionals in the accounting field. They apply their skills and work with accounting principles generally accepted, and other methods for managing finance. They also make use of the same types of records and systems for good reports. However, there is a specific challenge affecting medical accountants: the type of industry where the skills are applied.

The Health Care Compliance Association (HCCA) shows how medical accounting intertwines with a network of stakeholders, such as; patients, healthcare workers, medical facilities, insurance companies, pharmaceutical companies, device manufacturers for the medical field, employees and employers, government agencies. The result is, more complicated accounts to work on as a medical accountant.

Another difference, although a slight one, focuses on how payments in the healthcare system are dealt with. Payments for services rendered can be different from what is charged by the hospital. The complexity surrounding this payment system can be one tough nut to crack, thereby adding more difficulty to the challenging role of a medical accountant. Two different parties usually make the payments: insurance companies and the patients. The insurance company or provider can be privately owned or controlled by the government, as in the case of Medicare and Medicaid. They contribute payments on what is already negotiated. Payments done by patients are usually in copay, deductible, and coinsurance formats. The option of making payments from a healthcare savings account is also available.

Also, what is greatly considered important is the organization's decisions regarding finance. However, the role of a medical accountant still varies as there are other important concerns befitting to be considered: ensuring great quality services, due compensation for workers in the healthcare sector, targeting and improving the profit margin to go about carrying out these tasks.

For an ordinary accounting firm, where the sole aim is to amass good profits, the medical accountant is responsible for becoming aware of the above concerns. The lack of a good accounting team will cause damages to a healthcare system as such will find it difficult to get more medical personnel, provide professional and adequate care to patients, and manage the entire system cost-effectively. Healthcare fraud is also a rampant occurrence; hence, the role of a medical accountant will prove valuable.

Job Coding Prospects

The job of medical coding comes with lots of prospects and has, for quite some time, become one of the

high-valued and well-sought professions, giving exposure to so many job opportunities and hitting great
peaks in career growth. A good understanding of medical codes, policies covering payments, and various
government regulations, see medical coders transform
medical records into appropriate codes for billing and
insurance.

The roles of medical billers and coders in a healthcare
system have been known to be important. The usage of
electronic healthcare records (EHR) by medical facilities
and offices is on the rise; therefore, the services of medical billers and coders are needed to enter information
accurately, as they are well qualified to make use of
the technology. A good system with this approach will
provide great services to patients and ensure proper
payments of healthcare workers for services provided.

It is ideal you get to know the career prospects or out-
look in years to come. You may be curious about these
job roles and how easy it will be to get a job after spend-
ing time in school or if organizations are in high demand
for medical coders and billers.

Most jobs in the healthcare line are thriving, especially
that of medical billing and coding. As stated earlier,

the Bureau of Labour Statistics (BLS) projected a 22% increase in gainful employments of medical secretaries, such as professional billers and coders, by 2026. The projected rate is much faster when compared to rates given for other jobs. This sees a huge amount of job openings, about 129 000, being available in years to come.

Medical billing and coding are good jobs to be considered if you're so keen on job prospects or available job openings in the coming years, especially when searching for a good career. The number of aged individuals will increase with time and more medical care needed. For providing care and other medical services, there will be a need to update patients' medical records and a high rate in processing insurance claims. Regular healthcare claims will lead to an increase in demand for your skills, especially if you are into medical billing and coding. To appropriately process medical claims, the data required will need the services of a professional to get it organized and coded.

After acquiring the required level of training and being certified as a medical biller and coder, entry-level positions within this field are available to give a trial. Taking this and going further, the acquired experience can help you grow your career in healthcare, get more certifications, further your education, and other benefits.

Being a medical biller and coder offers you the opportunity to apply your skills in the following sectors, as most facilities, especially those in the medical field, which see, diagnose, and treat patients, need such services.

Hospitals

Medical laboratories Insurance companies Medical offices

Nursing homes Dental clinics Rehab clinics

Chapter 3: What Are The Medical Billing And Coding Classes Required?

The hospital is a setting where patients' good health is a top priority, and those at the helms of affairs commonly seen are usually the doctors, nurses, pharmacists, and lab scientists. Still, there are other professionals behind the scene whose collaborative efforts help keep things in order. These other professionals include medical billers and coders. They usually ensure proper channeling and communication between healthcare workers, patients, and insurance companies. Accurate documentation and processing of critical information are not left out. Doing all these promotes good reimbursement for services and treatments rendered, definitely fueling the zeal of healthcare workers to do more.

Classes usually focused on medical billing and coding are on various subjects that help interested students get the hang on managing medical records, codes application, submitting invoices, and provides any other form of assistance that can benefit the healthcare system.

Typical coursework for medical billing and coding includes technical knowledge, healthcare information, topics on business, all in a mix. Terminologies in the medical field are not left out as students will get to learn them, together with the cycle of healthcare claims and medical coding systems. Combining these subjects will serve as a good ground for getting the basics needed to advance in medical billing and coding, career-wise.

Some common courses associated with medical billing and coding includes:

- Diagnostic Coding

- Procedural Coding

- Billing and Coding Application

- Introduction to Computers

- Introduction to Healthcare Communication

- Medical Terminology

- Medical Law and Ethics

- Records Management

- Healthcare Settings, Claim Cycle, and Claims Processing

- Anatomy, Physiology, and Pathophysiology

The career path taken to be a medical biller and coder, compared to becoming a doctor, nurse, and any other healthcare professional, is less tasking and faster. A year or less is enough to get you started or make a switch to becoming a medical biller or coder.

There are tons of options available to choose from when settling on a career in this field. It is not a must to possess a bachelor's degree or have a two-year associate degree, seen with some billers and coders. There are various schools offering diplomas, certificates, and degree programs in medical billing and coding.

Medical Billing and Coding: Core Curriculum

Various courses in the field of medical billing and coding cover topics in clinical and clerical areas. The students are well taught on terminologies in anatomy, pharmacology, and other medical aspects. These courses are then effectively combined with others centering on business that deals with the management of records. It is imperative for professionals in this field to be abreast with the latest changes and trends in the healthcare sector, especially those on insurance billing and privacy laws.

Some essential medical billing and coding classes offered are:

Medical Terminology

The medical field has many terms or jargon that can be quite difficult to process on first contact, especially when one is not in the medical line. These jargons seem like an entirely different language. Some good examples are names or diagnoses given to diseases, medical codes written in shorthand, and treatment procedures.

This course exposes students to the origin of these terminologies and how they can be formed, defined, and analyzed.

Pharmacology

The world of pharmacology creates exposure to drugs and everything related. Drugs can serve a good purpose in the body system as well as cause dangers if not properly used or applied. It is quite important that administering a drug should go along with the correct name of the drug, its dosage, route, and any other information attached to the label or chart, as drugs with good healing potency can become toxic with wrong administration.

Pharmacology helps students learn different drug names, both the generic and trade names, how drugs work, side effects, contraindications, and interactions.

Body Systems 1 & 2

This class is in series, and students get to learn, practically, the human system, how they are structured, and the various functions they carry out. Students also get to understand the various medical terms associated with such systems. Some body systems include nervous, cardiovascular, digestive, musculoskeletal, respiratory systems.

The second series continues the first as it builds on it, giving more explorations on complex body systems and related terms.

Medical Office Procedures

This course offers students the required experience on everyday administrative assistant activities such as writing business letters, telephone call management, electronic mail processing, planning of meetings and travel, task management, specifically designed for the medical field.

Medical Contracts, Ethics, and HIPAA

This course focuses majorly on managed care contracts, covered patient services, Preventive health services, as well as office visits. Other aspects include ethics, knowledge on protected health information and disclosure-under Health Insurance Portability and Accountability (HIPAA), electronic health record (EHR) incentives which is a category of Health Information Technology for Economic and Clinical Health (HITECH) Act.

Basic Coding Using ICD-9 and ICD-10

There's a shorthand form or code specially designed for a particular kind of disease, sickness, condition, and required treatment. With these codes, identification and tracking of services carried out by healthcare providers to patients are simplified. Not only that, processing claims by medical billers become swift. Students get to learn both ICD-9 and 10 forms of coding. Also, some areas require special coding techniques: cardiology, pathology, and laboratory procedures. These are taught to students in this course.

Medical Billing and Health Insurance

This course introduces the basics. It gives insight into healthcare reimbursement and how payments are made for various health insurance. There's great exposure to payment systems, fee schedules, internal audit methods, and procedures involving coding.

Intermediate Medical Coding

There's a buildup of previous coding skills in this course. Here, students learn the various applications of the CPT and ICD-10 system of classification for coding diagnoses and treatment procedures.

Advanced Medical Coding Scenarios

This is similar to intermediate coding, except that more classification systems are applied. Students are able to create codes for diagnosis with CPT, ICD-9, ICD-10, and HCPCS in this course. The previous courses, which are basic and intermediate, are expanded to help students grasp the interpretation of complex medical data forms. This course also prepares them for the CPC-A certificate examination.

Coding for Medical Office Applications

Students get to learn skills involved in appropriate completion of medical claims forms using manual or electronic means. The form, CMS-1500, is usually applied, especially for Medicare claims, and helps show reasons why claims forms are delayed when processed or outrightly rejected.

Medical Billing and Coding Education Options

Yes! Every act done or applied with medical billing and coding requires a great deal of precision, but getting to learn how to go about the processes seems easy. Many students get to develop their skills from on-site training or programs in community colleges. Others gained knowledge from online means. Successful graduates are being offered appropriate certifications at the completion of a course, which shows they've been well trained, having the necessary skills and knowledge.

Bachelor's Degree Programs

If there's a need for you to obtain a bachelor's degree before going for a career in medical billing and coding, a study of this- health information management or health care administration, is necessary. More so, completing general education requirements is required. This is an added class to the major ones.

Trying to grab a Bachelor of Science or Arts degree will require you to offer courses in general sciences or liberal art. With a Bachelor's degree, you can make applications to several fields in the healthcare sector.

Prerequisites

A successful bachelor's degree program will need a high school diploma or GED and ACT or SAT, that is, after obtaining the required scores for the exams. There may also be inclusion of answers to essay questions, recommendations, and conducted interview sessions for possible admissions.

Courses

Courses for this degree program include health information management, medical terminologies, healthcare delivery systems, healthcare reimbursement, anatomy, pharmacology, physiology, and others.

Considerations

It is possible you want to delve into management positions as you proceed. Well, having a bachelor's degree will go a long way. Basic experience, as in the case of an internship, is one good requirement for a bachelor's degree.

Degree duration

It takes four years to attain this degree.

Certificate and Diploma Programs

These programs have a duration of 9 months to a year. There are various institutions of study offering these: career colleges, community colleges, professional organizations, and some other standalone programs. The duration to complete a program in career colleges can be quite lesser.

Prerequisites

This can be the same as a Bachelor's degree program: having a high school diploma or GED, passing or getting the required scores for tests such as ACT or SAT.

Courses

You get to study anatomy and physiology, patient privacy, medical terminologies, classification of diseases, and coding techniques.

Considerations

Get to know the type of coding system that is applicable in the program. It is possible some programs delve into hospital coding systems or office coding.

Degree duration

It ranges from 9 months to a year.

Associate Degree Programs

When compared with certificate or diploma programs on medical billing and coding, associate degrees take longer to complete. What is being studied is way more than just what is needed to be known in medical billing and coding careers. Career and community colleges are very much available to offer you this degree program.

Prerequisites

You need a high school diploma or GED and a good grade point average (GPA) of 2.0 or above. Some programs may require coursework done beforehand, like anatomy and physiology.

Courses

Courses include diagnostic coding skills, procedural coding, ethics, medical terminologies, pharmacology.

Considerations

Having a plan to delve higher into the educational ladder by obtaining a bachelor's degree or master's, may require a transfer of credits from your associate degree.

Degree duration

Associate degree programs take two years to complete.

Online Colleges

Following up with online courses on medical billing and coding may take up to ten months to round up and at an affordable fee. Two things are important requirements to ease your way through with study: a good computer system and internet access. You can also get to buy other helpful course materials online. A decision can come up from faculty boards or members to improve study with videos, virtual labs, articles, and work simulations. These online colleges can also prop you up for major certification examinations on coding.

Recently, certificates, diplomas, Bachelor's degrees, and associate programs are springing up online. This is quite beneficial for those finding it very difficult to get used to the traditional methods these programs use.

Online means of study and traditional methods produce the same result; that is, they both give the required knowledge on the needed basics and equip you with the necessary coding skills. The major difference between these methods is flexibility. Online courses are much more flexible; that's why they are in high demand these days among students who work and study alongside, or have other important responsibilities.

Online courses and programs have a way of introducing you to the basics and what medical billing and coding entail before going ahead to invest all necessary resources, time, and money inclusive, in obtaining a degree or certificate.

Certification and Certifying Bodies

Getting certified brings important recognition. After bagging your degree or rounding up a particular medical billing and coding program, there are available opportunities for you to get good certifications. Certifications can be of two kinds: general or specific, and it boils down to the kind of specialty you want. General certification is getting certified in foundational coding, while specific has to do with narrowing or niching down to a particular topic like anesthesia or obstetrics and gynecology. Having a specific certification shows you off as someone who is an expert in that field.

Several bodies offer certifications in medical billing and coding. One of such is the American Academy of Professional Coders (AAPC) which offers a certificate of Certified Professional Coder (CPC). Attaining this certificate gives you a vast level of recognition in physician's office settings. It sees you as a specialist in the world of medical coding, with vast knowledge and experience. Certification can also be gotten in other areas dealing with in-patient and out- patient coding techniques and risk adjustment.

Another example of a certificate offering body is the American Health Information Management Association (AHIMA). This body offers certificates like Certified Coding Associate (CCA), showing good proficiency in medical coding. The CCA is given especially to individuals with all qualifications to render services in different settings like hospitals or private practices. Those who render services in one setting are offered certificates also.

Deciding on the Right Educational Track

You've decided to become a medical biller or coder, but what serves as a challenge is the right path to follow in making choices on a particular program. One thing to consider is the nature of flexibility. Ask yourself if it is flexible as some programs have a better degree of flexibility than others do. Can you cope well as you tend to balance your studies with other responsibilities like work, family life, and others? You can also make inquiries if there is a part-time program or available pre-recorded classes for your convenience.

Another factor is the preference of medical setting. Different coding systems are available and applied more in the hospital setting or physician's office. If you've chosen the particular route, ensure there's an available program taking that coding system.

Getting a job in urban settings can probably get you a higher paycheck than jobs in rural areas but can be very competitive to get. Well, acquiring more educational levels and training can avail you of opportunities to apply for regular jobs.

Chapter 4: What Does A Specialist In Medical Billing And Coding Do?

Being a medical biller and coder comes with its assigned tasks. As well, you, being a professional in this field, get a wide range of opportunities to offer your services in one of the most thriving occupations. These professionals are part of the medical secretaries under the Bureau of Labor Statistics (BLS). As known, projected a 22% rise in employment opportunities between 2016 and 2026, amounting to 129000 job opportunities. The need for the services of a medical biller or coder will increase as the population is aging, with more need for healthcare services.

Medical billing and coding professionals are part of the team working behind effortlessly to see to the smooth running of the industry. They help set up a direct link between services rendered by healthcare providers and appropriate reimbursement. In terms of educational requirements and training, medical billers and coders require less when compared with other professionals in the medical world, but their importance should not be written off as they are key to a medical organization being successful.

There's a need for an appointed person or professional to take up the job of medical billing and coding for insurance and invoice for patients. Doctors or office managers have their specific responsibilities in the hospital setting. Still, they may also take up the billing and coding job or get more staff to take it up. Healthcare providers are more focused on the patients, so taking responsibility for the billing and coding job can be difficult; hence, jobs are assigned to specialists in the field. They oversee administrative works involving coding and billing to ensure proper reimbursement of healthcare providers.

Medical coders can niche down to become an expert in a particular aspect of coding, for example, a specialist in cancer treatment. The sole responsibility of a medical coding professional is to create appropriate codes for every diagnosis and treatment rendered. The coding system operates in such a way that it follows up the diagnosis and treatment of patients, thereafter placing them into a diagnosis- related group (DRG). Medicare and health insurance programs apply this system of coding for reimbursement of rendered services.

Professional billers and coders work, on a typical day, in an office environment, having a total of 40 hours per workweek. Some hospitals run a 24-hour health infor-mation department, and they have coding professionals who are available to work at night and during weekends.

It is imperative to have medical billers and coders in every sector of healthcare. They make sure health-relat-ed data are well organized and readily available for use by personnel in the facility. These coders and billers cre-ate a link and act as an intermediate between medical offices and insurance companies; they make it easy for medical facilities to process insurance claims, invoices, and make payments. Work entails the usage of electronic data at most times, but on the other hand, some offices do make use of paper files. This clearly means that having good computer skills is one requirement of a medical biller and coder as most jobs are processed electronically.

An intricate part of this job is precision and accuracy. All jobs involving billing and coding have to be done accurately. Using the correct data will ensure patients get the care they need and the insurance company receives the right information to process claims and reimburse them.

More so, patients' vital information can be compromised if not well handled. It is the responsibility of medical billers and coders to protect patients' data at all times adequately. The law system has enforced confidentiality of patients. Therefore, there must be enhanced security measures on all data being dealt with.

Having good knowledge of classification systems is one important requirement for a medical billing and coding professional. A professional makes use of these universal codes to organize every information pertaining to a patient. This knowledge is applied in such a way that healthcare providers get reimbursed for services rendered and other medical procedures carried out by insurance companies. The codes, also, are used as standard forms of patients' medical histories and treatment information records. This process makes things easier even when there are various medical specialists attending to patients in terms of making diagnoses and providing treatments.

Medical Coding

A specialist in medical coding kickstarts the day by going through reports that need to be coded. It is a direct job, no complexities. Here, the coder gets the report detailing a procedure or checkup by the doctor, goes through it, and then decides on the appropriate way to get the information translated into codes.

An example can be in the form of a complaint of sore throat by a patient, written by the doctor, during the visit. The doctor then examines the area and suspects an infection caused by streptococcus, commonly affecting the throat. A test for streptococcus is then performed. After confirmation of the presence of the infection, the doctor diagnoses a case of strep throat and prescribes a drug, amoxicillin, an antibiotic, to be taken. The coder gets hold of this information, and after taking a read, applies the ICD- 10-CM and CPT codes from the manual. This is after making a decision on the best coding method for the diagnosis and treatment process. For the above example, a CPT code of 87880 is applicable for the strep test carried out, 00781-6041 for prescribed medications, in this case, amoxicillin, and ICD-10-CM code J02. 0, for the diagnosis of streptococcal sore throat.

After determining the codes, the coder inputs them correctly into a particular form, enters them into a computer program, and then takes up the next report. These processes: going through the reports, making decisions on appropriate codes and translation of reports, inputting codes into forms, cover the entire day. Coding is straightforward, so with time, a coder gets used to applicable codes for procedures that are very much common in the office. For example, code application for general office visit, 99214, and flu shots, 90657, are easily remembered by a coder for a general practitioner as they get used to the system. Note that there are guidelines for every code, and coders must follow such. One is proper code order for certain conditions.

In all these, cases may arise where there seems to be a sort of confusion or codes coming down with gray areas, and guidelines to be applied getting too complex, maybe due to the symptoms, diagnosis, or treatment procedures becoming too advanced and complicated. It may become possible that no solution is seen in the appropriate manuals or guidelines. Well, a good resort, by most coders, will be to seek out advice and guidance from other coding communities.

One thing that a coder must be sure of is correspondence between the procedure code and diagnosis code. This is imperative. If there's no correspondence existing between the listed procedure and diagnosis, the processed claim may be rejected, thereby affecting the reimbursement for provided services.

Another good consideration is lag time for coding reports. Each office possesses this, specifically, and it lasts between two to five working days. Coding processes ought to be completed within this period, five days of the patient's hospital visit. Working with these deadlines promotes the smooth running of the reimbursement process. The coder has a huge role to play in working and meeting up with the deadline.

Medical Billing

A medical biller begins operations as soon as the medical coder completes work. It's the medical biller's obligation to make precise, lawful bills for the healthcare provider's office and have them delivered quickly to an insurance agency or payer. The biller must also convey and receive the payments from patients. What follows is a shortened portrayal of the medical charging process.

The medical biller's day includes various activities. The biller is liable for making accurate and officially right claims, checking for exactness in transaction reports and making bills for patients.

The road to all these processes starts when the biller has access to the codes created by the medical coder. The codes may be in either form or electronic formats, that is, computer programs. From this, a medical claim is made. A claim contains a list of all procedures, services rendered, and the appropriate costs, from the healthcare provider to the patients, for collection of reimbursement. This is the summary of the whole process. It seems quite easy from what is explained but, it can be very much complicated.

It starts off with correspondence. The medical biller makes sure all codes correspond. This is one necessary check after the coder has completed the task of translation. The medical biller handling such a task must have good knowledge of medical terminology and be up to date with the current CPT, ICD, and HCPCS codes.

Another good check is familiarity with the insurance policy of patients. A medical biller must have this knowledge to make sure that the patients' plan covers the services and procedures carried out by the healthcare worker. Every service, procedure, and corresponding code, listed on the claim should be billable. This is what the medical coder should make sure of. Well, everything rests in the hands of the payer, and the agreed contract between either patient or healthcare worker has with the payer. Under the policy holder's contract, insurance payers put forth rules serving as guidelines to what attracts billing and what doesn't.

Same way insurance payers have their rules, so also, medical facilities have their own rates for every procedure or service. With this, a medical biller will know how to make a claim that goes along with the facility's rate. These factors are considered when making an accurate medical claim. On completion of the claim, the medical biller sends it to the payer. It is possible the claim doesn't go directly to the payer but first, through a clearinghouse. It all depends on the type of payer receiving the claim. Also, note that some payers and clearinghouses make use of software or special forms.

After the payer has successfully received a claim, an evaluation is done on it. This is referred to as payer adjudication. The payer then makes a decision on the amount payable to the healthcare provider as reimbursement. This is sent back to the healthcare provider as a transaction report. Such a report gets to the medical biller, who then provides proper review and accuracy checks. What is being checked for is the correspondence between the charges and what was established between the healthcare provider and payer. To confirm the accuracy, the medical biller prepares a payment bill for the patient, giving an explanation in the process, on covered services and procedures, actual procedure being paid for, and the cost of payment.

A medical biller's day on the job starts to end with collections. Some patients may find it difficult to make payment, or others not showing any willingness to pay for services. The medical biller then has a duty to send appropriate reminders to such patients. If there is no response, the bills are sent to a collections service as a last resort. These services are tasked differently, depending on the policy established by the healthcare provider.

Can One Person Take Up Both Jobs?

Most times, the roles of a medical biller and coder are assigned to different employees, but some cases see both jobs done by a person. Facilities with a small organizational structure, like a standalone office, may employ someone with both billing and coding skills. It can be that the hiring market is quite small, so candidates who are proficient in both positions are usually preferred. For a much larger organization, like hospitals and health systems, the job roles are usually for different experts. The division of both roles is more sensible from a financial perspective. This is in the sense that medical billers are less paid than coders. Well, this doesn't necessarily mean that medical coders shouldn't have good knowledge of billing. A good certification in medical coding can broaden the edge to change careers and get good pay.

Summary of the Job Duties for Medical Billing and Coding Specialists

This summarizes the daily activities of a medical biller and coder. Note that some tasks vary, and this depends on what the employer needs.

- Ensure the proper organization of data at all times.

- Prompt review of medical reports.

- See to complete and accurate medical records.

- Enter the corresponding codes into the medical software for proper reimbursement of healthcare providers and patients.

- Proper follow-up of patients' outcomes for assessment of quality.

- Use the correct format when entering healthcare records for medical registries.

- Confidentiality of patients' information is strictly adhered to.

- Maintenance of good electronic records. This is

to allow medical personnel to retrieve, analyze, and make reports on data when appropriate.

- Applying the appropriate codes when a patient is fully diagnosed to help in proper administration of care and help health statisticians to track population data.

- Carry out extensive reviews on patients' medical records to ensure correct data coding for previous services.

- Established as a link between the medical facility and an insurance company.

Chapter 5: How To Become A Medical Biller And Coder?

The skills of medical billing and coding are in high demand. One way to become one, and proven to be effective, is going through the required training. Well, with on-the-job experience, you can delve into this field, but some job specifications for a particular position require specialized education, which usually varies for different employers.

Claiming the title of a medical biller or coder allows you to take a path possessing few options in the education line. One notable fast route is obtaining a certificate or doing a diploma program, which is more often less than one year. Pursuing a degree is another good alternative. A degree program can be the best bet in getting positions where requirements are quite strict. Getting an associate degree involves taking classes in general education and other coursework on healthcare, billing, and coding. The duration for completing this program is usually two years. As for Certifications, they are not left out as some employers usually ask for them.

As a professional medical biller or coder, it is a necessity that you possess good knowledge of various medical codes, policies involving payments, and government regulations. A good understanding of job requirements about this field prepares one for what is ahead before diving in, and not only that, a swipe at succeeding in this field needs the necessary skills and knowledge, and that can take some time. Being in possession of analytical and organizational skills and attention to detail can help a great deal in succeeding as a medical biller and coder.

In making decisions about the best available education option, one thing should be in mind, and that is, your chosen career plan. The employment process and requirements by employers come in different ways, with various requirements. Ensure you go through these requirements when checking for openings in these orga-nizations where your preference is direct.

You may have the interest to go into management-level roles, like a thought for the future. Not bad. Associate degrees are there to give you an edge. If you eventually decide to go further in education to advance in career levels, earned credits in an associate degree could be transferred, possibly, into a bachelor's degree program. The transfer can be on the ground where your institution of study partners with other institutions that have agreed to accept the earned credits for a bachelor's degree program.

Becoming a Medical Coder

The role of a medical coder is one required field in the healthcare sector, offering great service behind the scenes. This field is growing rapidly, and it is best suitable for one with a desire to work in positions where there's no direct or face-to-face contact with patients. Being well detail-oriented and having specialized skills are significant requirements.

Getting acquainted with this job role is pretty much easy. What you need is either an associate or bachelor's degree that is science- related and other credentials. The below steps serve as a guide to becoming a medical coder.

Get a Post-Secondary Education

Acquiring a degree after secondary education is not needed to grab the title of a medical coder, but some job specifications usually hit on having a prerequisite education, especially as applicants. There are several available options like bachelor's and associate degrees, certificate programs. One best alternative is attending schools specially designed for medical coding or running an education program in that line.

It doesn't matter the kind of route you take to acquire post-secondary education for a medical coding career. Just make sure the program and institution running it, is well recognized or accredited. Three bodies are directly involved in the accreditation of specific programs in medical coding - the American Health Informatics Management Association (AHIMA), the American Association of Professional

Coders (AAPC), and the Commission on Accreditation for Health Informatics and Information Management Education (CAHIIM).

Get Preliminary Credentials

All medical coding program types require certifications that can be acquired after writing the basic exams for such credentials.

A good example of one, which can also be touted as a first option, is Certified Coding Associate (CCA). This certification is widely recognized nationally and seen as a standard of achievement based on health information management. The body controlling this certification, AHIMA, gave recommendations on possessing work experience of about six months before taking the certification examination. For applicants who have rounded up a program approved by AHIMA, or any other program centered on medical coding, there's no need to have any work experience.

Another option is a certification by Registered Health Information Technician (RHIT). Having work experience beforehand isn't quite a requirement, but it specifies a need to possess associate-level health information and management knowledge obtained from a program accredited by CAHIIM.

Work Experience

After bagging that degree or being certified as a medical coder, it's now time to actually know what it feels like to work in this field. You're now certified and want to practice. Some useful resources while in school or networking amongst friends and colleagues can help when seeking a job. AHIMA and the AAPC are associations you can be a part of as you're more likely to be well exposed to several employment opportunities and resources for career development.

Being on the job and acquiring experience builds you as a professional. Not only that, you'll get to learn more about your job preferences like work setting, either hospital-based or practicing in a physician environment. This will also help you focus on the proper certification to acquire for further career advancement.

Advanced Medical Coding Certifications

You've gained some level of work experience. Now you have the opportunity to obtain further professional certifications. These available certifications from AHIMA include Certified Coding Specialist (CCS) or the Certified Coding Specialist Physician-Based (CCS-P) certificates.

Certified Coding Specialist certificate is for professional coders with skills based on the classification of patients' medical records in a hospital setting. It further tests your knowledge in medical terminology, disease processes, pharmacology, experience in ICD- 10-CM and CPT or HCPCS coding systems.

The Certified Coding Specialist Physician-Based certificate shows that a professional coder is certified to work in a physician-based setting. The examination tests your mastery-level understanding of ICD-10-CM, HCPCS (Level 2), and CPT coding systems. It tests at advanced level and not necessarily entry-level skills.

Career Advancement

There's an opportunity for career advancement even after obtaining an advanced level of certification. You can keep on practicing as a medical coder while seeking out means to further your career. Advancing your career can be of several forms: taking up leadership positions like managerial roles, compliance auditor, consultant, or possibly, going for advanced education.

Becoming a Medical Biller

The thoughts of being a medical biller can be brought to life even while still in high school. Courses that can put you in line of study are English, biology, communications, computer science, chemistry, and mathematics. On obtaining your high school diploma, proceed to an associate degree program accredited by Accreditation for Health Informatics and Information Management Education.

Going through a program under an associate degree puts you on a way of understanding medical billing as a field. It helps you gain the necessary skills to attain a successful career. You can either go further to get a bachelor's degree or seek employment opportunities.

A bachelor's degree program explores different aspects of business and health care. You can as well go further in related educational programs which are very much higher or get employed. Degrees in health informatics, healthcare administration, and information management are done by many to break into administrative or supervisory works.

On your own volition, you can acquire certification and further your education in the course of advancing your career. This will avail you the opportunity to remain up-to-date with changes or trends in software applications, technological advancement, and occupational ethics. AHIMA offers these certifications and education. At the end of the program, an examination is to be written which confers the certification.

Chapter 6: What Are Your Qualifications As A Specialist In Medical Billing And Coding?

The roles of a medical biller and coder in an organization are different, with different requirements or specifications, based on what the employer is looking for. A whole lot of employers ask for a certificate, diploma, or associate degree when seeking a professional medical biller and coder. Another common one is industry certification.

Certification in line with medical billing and coding officially recognizes you as an expert in that field. A great achievement indeed. Sometimes, these certificates may not be needed. On the other hand, some states demand them. Candidates who are certified stand a better chance of getting a job than those without one or two certifications by some employers' standards.

A certificate in medical billing and coding offers you opportunities to venture into high-demand professions. A medical biller and coder work together to

There's a high chance of being successful in the world of medical billing and coding when you've earned your qualifications or are fully certified. Certification is done by a body well recognized and trusted, such as the American Association of Professional Coders (AAPC) or American Health Information Management Association (AHIMA). They are considered the primary credentialing bodies. These two bodies have different modes of operations and unique standards applicable to obtaining their certifications. Certificates offered by AHIMA are based on coding in hospitals, while that of AAPC cover other personnel.

The certifications these bodies offer come with good benefits, and that depends on how you want to apply them during career advancement. Some certifications create opportunities for work in a hospital setting or prepare you for a role in a physicians' office. Be aware that certain training programs usually go with certain forms of certifications. When deciding on the type of certification you really want before you go all out, put this in mind.

Certification Organizations

American Association of Professional Coders (AAPC)

The American Association of Professional Coders was founded officially in 1988 with two objectives: providing educational services and certifications to qualified medical coders practicing in physicians' offices and putting great standards of coding into place by working with already accepted standards.

The organization's initial goal was to raise the standards pertaining to outpatient medical coding, but present standards on certifications and training have been raised. This training now covers every aspect of the healthcare sector. One can now be certified in medical coding, medical billing, auditing, compliance, medical documentation, and practice management. As a member, there's a mandatory yearly payment of member-ship fee, which costs $180, but it comes at a reduced cost for students with good proof of an active student, which is $100.

American Health Information Management Association (AHIMA)

Certifications by AHIMA focus mainly on coders in hospital settings. This organization was founded in 1928 with a goal, at the initial stage, to ensure improvement in the quality of medical records. Still, it is obligated to attain excellence in the integrity of medical records using electronic medical records.

The organization offers several training programs, holds conventions yearly, and organizes workshops in different areas for several days. AHIMA makes it possible to gain access to huge resources, training, and lots of opportunities to network during your career. One difference between AHIMA and AAPC is that it offers entry-level certifications as opposed to AAPC, which offers apprentice-level certifications. If you've had good experience in medical coding, then AHIMA certifications are well suited for you.

To be a member of this organization, a payment of $135 is to be made yearly. That's the standard payment. For students, it comes at a reduced fee, about $49, yearly. For first-timers, they are to pay the sum of $79, while older members of 65 years and above pay $49. Costs for certification examinations are offered at a discount to approved members.

Medical Billing Certifications

A certified medical biller depicts one as having the expertise to deal effectively with every aspect of medical billing with any form of compromise on the process of reimbursement. The well-known and approved certification for medical billers is the certified professional biller (CPB).

The certified professional biller (CPB) qualification shows a good level of proficiency in medical billing formalities and reimbursement cycle, preparation and submission of appeals where there's denial, preauthorization, posting of payments, and proper follow up on issues concerning outstanding fees. They possess the right skills with broad experience to steer an organization in the right direction, promote the smooth running of operations, and proper financial management of medical practices and organizations.

The examination for CPB tests applicants on insurance requirements and how private insurance is different from public health plans, managed care, and worker's compensation. A certified holder has knowledge of best coding practices, both local or national coverage and the guidelines covering them, and government policies on healthcare and debt collection.

Certification Requirements

The AAPC considers two requirements: recent member-ship for CPB and possession of an associate degree, at least. Interested applicants for the certificate should be well prepared for the exam, taking into considera-tion the various components, with special attention to Health Insurance Portability and Accountability or False Claims Act.

Medical Coding Certification

As a certified medical coder, you have gained a level of knowledge in various codes identifying medical ser-vices rendered, the procedures, and supplies for billing purposes and reimbursement. There are guidelines that cover coding practices, and as a certified coder, you have knowledge on how such should be applied using resources like CPT, ICD, and HCPCS. Code sets can become obsolete with time, so they are regularly updated. This implies continuous education and training programs to enable coders to keep up with updates in coding systems, thus maintaining their professionalism.

Some medical coding certifications are:

Certified Coding Associate (CCA)

This certification is given to medical coders who can perform operations in various settings such as hospitals and physicians' offices.

Correct Coding Specialists (CCS)

A specialist with this certificate possesses the ability to organize data of inpatient or outpatient in a hospital. This certification shows you have great expertise in diagnosis and procedural coding, a level that can be way more than the CCA. The CCS is mainly offered by the AHIMA.

A certified CCS holder also has experience in both Current Procedural Terminology (CPT) and International Classification of

Diseases (ICD) coding systems.

Correct Coding Specialist-Physician Based (CCS-P)

This certifies you to work in physician settings, group practices, and specialized clinics, with the responsibility of assigning ICD-10 diagnostic codes and CPT procedural codes to medical records. You possess a great deal of knowledge in health information and are subject to data quality.

Certified Inpatient Coder (CIC)

This coder deals with inpatient records and facility coding. Specialists have the ability to make correct inpatient codes from existing medical records and have an understanding of how outpatient reimbursement processes work.

Certified Outpatient Coding (COC)

Being a COC holder means you are proficient in applying the correct codes for diagnosis, procedures, and other services done in outpatient settings. Also, applicable for coding emergency department visits, same-day surg-eries, physical or speech therapy.

Certified Professional Coder (CPC)

This certification is widely recognized and shows you, a holder, as someone with a good level of training and experience. You are proficient in observing and tak-ing readings from medical charts and applying correct codes using ICD, CPT, and HCPCS coding systems.

Certified Professional Coder- Payer (CPC-P)

This applies to coders who practice in organizations dealing with medical claims for payment. Skills usually focus on claims already delivered to private or public health plans such as Medicare or Medicaid. The exami-nation tests you on adjudication of claims from the per-spective of the payer, the differences between process-es assigned to a healthcare provider and the insurance company.

Certified Risk Adjustment Coder (CRAC)

Competent skills include interpretation of medical charts and application of appropriate codes in risk ad-justment models. Certified coders have in-depth knowledge of compliance, reimbursement, and processes involving audits.

How Important Are Certifications

You can go into other aspects of medical billing and coding or evolve, career wise, without the need for a certificate, but having one shows your level of competence and knowledge in the field. Certifications are quite important, and it does you no harm or disadvantage to get one. Here are some reasons:

Earning a Decent Pay

As noted by the American Academy of Professional Coders (AAPC), a body in charge of certifications, having a certificate or multiple certifications in the field of medical billing and coding creates an avenue to earn above-average pay. You have even more chances with multiple certifications than those with only one qualification. A certificate holder earns an average of $55,960 compared to those with different certifications, with earnings amounting to $65,000.

Professional Connections

Interested coders on the lookout for certifications can be a part of organizations in charge of certifications without necessarily possessing one. Being a member can avail you of opportunities to connect with other professionals in the field. Other professionals are like minds who place great value on professional certifications and education. This is an exposure to amazing career opportunities.

Good Employability Status

It has been well established that the medical billing and coding field has a projected growth of 22% through 2026. This projection was made by the Bureau of Labor Statistics. There's a telling difference in the rate of growth when compared to other occupations, given the percentage. Of course, the rate places the employment level in an advantageous position, but the market is still competitive. With a certificate in hand, you have a good chance of getting employment.

Personal Growth and Development

You feel a certain level of achievement having aced a certification examination. Yes! Not only for potential employers, but yourself. You develop confidence in the work you put in, and with further training come improved knowledge and growth levels as a professional.

Medical Billing and Coding Skills

Aside from going through rigorous training and programs, a professional medical biller and coder should possess the necessary skills to carry out every assigned role. These skills can sometimes be what employers look for in a job seeker. Some important skills appropriate for medical billing and coding include:

Good attention to details

One very important quality to possess as you'll be dealing with a range of digits from five to six digit numbers, especially for medical coders. The coding systems are mostly numbers, so you'll need focus and eyes to spot errors easily. Poor attention to important details can mark works, which is equivalent to more rejected claims.

Computer proficiency

A good medical biller and coder should possess computer skills as major billing activities are done digitally as opposed to the system of using paper. It will be very easy to deal with billing and coding tasks appropriately if you're good with the computer.

Bookkeeping

For medical billers, knowledge of bookkeeping basics will help link statements with that of payments. This is for insurer's process claims. It is not necessary to attain training in advanced accounting skills for bookkeeping skills.

Organizational skills

As a medical biller and coder, you'll attend to different types of forms for patients, and they are to be correctly completed. Improper arrangements or disorganized presentations of forms can hamper work progress.

Confidentiality skills

Healthcare information, especially that of patients, must be kept or well secured from the outside world. The HIPAA laws mandate confidentiality of patients' vital information at all times, except in obtaining payer reimbursement. Privacy is to be respected. Also, improper discussions on patients' details amongst colleagues are not encouraged, except with those still in such cases.

Data analysis

This skill involves making quick decisions and assessments on coming across various codes in groups to make sure they are appropriate based on what is on the patient's record. You should also be able to correct spotted errors when analyzing data.

Teamwork and collaborative skill

A professional medical biller and coder will constantly communicate with colleagues, patients, medical officers, and insurance companies regularly. It is important to collaborate well with other members to promote the smooth running of the facility.

This can also be in line with possessing good and strong communication skills.

Compassion and sensitivity

You'll be dealing with patients on activities involving claims, although, not in all cases. In such situations, a good sense of compassion, being well sensitive and patient, will go a long way in patient management.

Adaptability

One skill you need to possess as a medical biller and coder is blending with new systems. There's constant upgrade and integration of brand new software, technological advancement, and improved standards of practice in the medical world, affecting billing standards - all in the billing and coding sector. As a professional in the field, you must be willing to fit in with new developments.

Chapter 7: How To Select And Prepare For Certification Medical Code?

One thing you'll certainly be doing as you go into the medical billing and coding field is making decisions and taking the right steps. Well, so it is whenever we want to go into something new. Do you want to choose a program or certification? Then, you need to take out time to weigh the available options and pick out the one that best suits your needs. A good start is by looking out for medical billing and coding jobs in your locality and observing the necessary qualifications demanded by employers.

Choosing the Appropriate Certification

Decision making on the right type of certification to build your career is a two-way thing. Take note of these factors when going for a certification:

The training program for that certification: can you balance your time with that of the program? Do you have a good budget? Is the curriculum sort of interesting?

Your long-term career goals: what role do you want to finally settle in as a professional? Do you have a particular facility or setting in mind? What activities do you want to be involved in to cover up your time?

The answers to all these questions can make it easy to focus on a certification that will benefit your career goals and education.

Considering the Educational Requirements

The requirements in earning a certification differ. Some certifications may require you to have earned a degree with four years of study before qualifying to take the exam. Others may demand for a short- term program. The American Health Information Management Association (AHIMA) and American Academy of Professional

Coders (AAPC) mandate interested applicants to have gone through a training program. These training programs, especially the accredited ones, put you on the line of getting trained and educated to practice in the healthcare sector and ace the exam. Online programs and vocational training are good examples of training options that can be considered.

One thing is, there are advantages and disadvantages to these programs, but take your mind off that. Important things to note are if such programs are accredited and if there's surety of getting well trained by the expertise of the instructors.

The kind of training offered by some schools are either focused based, that is, they teach what is available to specific certification, or focused on general education, providing general knowledge to write the certification examination. You won't be wrong in taking enough time to choose a good program that can set you on the right career path. That will definitely be a good head start. So, search within. Your guts can come in handy too. Go for what you feel is appropriate for your goals, style of learning, and schedules. If you take a look at your budget, schedules, means of learning, and they all suit the college program which covers the AHIMA educational needs, then go for that certification path. If the vocational school in your locality is accredited and bases its teaching on the AAPC program, you can follow that path also. In all, there's a good chance of getting gainfully employed in the end.

When you look at all available options on ground, just know that a good one well suited for medical billing and coding will prepare you adequately for entry-level certification.

The Decision to Pursue a Degree

Degree and certification types depend on the school offering such. An example is community colleges that offer associate degree programs. It is your responsibility to know what a program you're interested in offers and what degree you will be conferred with at the end of the study period.

Based on importance, an earned degree may not measure up to the certifications you want to specialize in, but getting one comes with lots of benefits. A degree increases the chances of earning decent pay. Some employers fancy having a degree that offers better pay incentives to potential employees with a degree and certificate. Some may wave off having a certificate as a professional coder, but certified coders have good wage potential. Also, a degree offers you more job opportunities.

Prioritizing your Career Needs

What is being considered in career advancement is long-term or future goals. The future can't be accurately predicted, at least not all the time. It is a good avenue to think about your career needs in the long run when making a pick on the training program available. A bad pick can affect your career in the future such as the chosen program, although it gets you prepared for a certification exam, but doesn't fit into your plan career-wise.

Some factors to consider when making this decision

Your preferred employment setting, such as a hospital, physician's office.

What job do you have in mind? Coding, billing, charge posting, or accounts receivable follow-up. Tilting towards the introverted personality and attention to detail are good fits for the role as a coder. They tend to work solely on their own. If you have the same personality trait, you may best fit in the role as a medical coder. This goes the same way with other roles that seek the right personality fit, like medical billing and charge posting. Someone who's on the go and very social may fit well into the account receivable follow-up because there's constant communication with individuals around, most likely payers.

The type of certification being demanded by potential employers.

The training program available. It's quality and cost.

Employability Demands

Choosing the kind of setting you want to work in and the particular job you're interested in will carry the bulk of your decision-making process. Of course, you want to see how you can raise your marketability standards and make yourself a good candidate for most jobs.

These are some good tips to know the basics of what potential employers require and what certifications are demanded.

Employment recruiters in your locality are good bets to get tips on what credentials are usually demanded.

Some medical offices display advertisements for job roles. Note the credentials.

Local job listings are also a good source. Take a look and observe the certificate requirements for jobs you're interested in.

If you've found an organization that catches your attention, be on the lookout for the quality of coders they seek. The organization may very well be interested in employing coders with certificates from AHIMA approved programs. Then, it will be good to go for such

approved programs or take an exam organized by the body. Suppose the same hospital or organization employs coders with AHIMA and AAPC certifications. In that case, it will be in your best interest to go for programs that will train you enough for the exams and expose you to seas of job opportunities.

Taking the Certification Exam

After selecting a training or certificate program and undergoing rigorous training for the required period, the next stage is attempting the medical billing and coding certification examination.

To take the certification exam, there are some prerequisites attached. After the required study periods, a major prerequisite for an exam is good knowledge in medical terminology; anatomy, ICD- 10, and CPT codify systems, reimbursement rules, and compliance. Accuracy and attention to detail are required skills for every medical biller and coder. You are required to make every activity or role involving numbers: procedure codes, diagnosis codes, insurance policy numbers, billing address, and other numbers involving activities- are accurate when they are prepared for reimbursement.

In addition, there are other prerequisites for the organizing bodies, AHIMA and AAPC.

Prerequisites for AHIMA Certification Examination

The American Health Information Management Association (AHIMA) is in charge of offering the following certifications: CCA, CCS, CCS-P. One of the most basic requirements for an entry-level certification is to possess a high school degree diploma or an equivalent before attempting the examination. For other levels, AHIMA demands a bachelor's degree or other higher ones to qualify for the certification examination. The available training programs for medical billing and coding do not have particular requirements for enrollment. You can get enrolled after finishing your high school program or graduating out from college. But it has been explained that the certifications examination requires some educational prerequisites. So, in the application process for a certification program, ensure you have all the requirements to qualify you for the exam.

Prerequisites for AAPC Certification Examination

The American Academy of Professional Coders (AAPC) offers CPC, COC, CPC-P, CIC certificates. There's no specification by AAPC on requiring a high school diploma or any equivalent, for enrolment, but it is deemed as what is recommended. In the same way, specialized certifications, as mandated by the AAPC, require a good level of experience in what you want to specialize in, before you can put in for that certification.

Preparing for the Certification Examination

The time for the examination is drawing nearer. You've undergone the training and have chosen the appropriate certification examination in line with your career goals. What is left is surmounting the exam, which requires a good amount of study time and adequate preparations. Here are some useful tips for gaining the most out of your study time.

Good Study Routine and Strategy

A good study technique will make preparations much easier. Hard work is key, but applying a bit of smart work will take a chunk of pressure off you as you prepare. You need a good understanding of what you're studying, especially when the materials are a lot. You can prioritize important materials during your study.

Study methods differ for every individual, well agreed, but some existing and proven techniques can offer a bit of ease in studying. One proven way to build retention is to go through the required material, give proper attention or listen attentively when discussions are ongoing, and put down what has been learned in your own words. You should know what kind of learner personality you have. Some people are so stimulated visually that they remember what has been seen. Some can retain what has been heard earlier, that is, auditory learning. Another category is those that can connect movement with various concepts. No matter what kind of learning method appeals to you, do a lot of practice on retaining information in ways that are very beneficial. You can practice using flashcards, videos, audios or podcasts, study notes, or whatever best suits you.

Setting up your Own Space

Utmost concentration is what is needed for a good study session. To prevent any disturbance, create a study space. It could be a quiet area in your home. These are helpful tips:

Pick a suitable area: the setting of study areas has a way of affecting your rate of assimilation. Some personalities fancy a classroom setting for the reason that it helps them study well. They set up a chair and a table in a particular area. Some take solace in curling up in a chair to study. It's risky, though, as one can easily fall asleep. So, make sure the chair isn't too comfortable.

Choose areas with fewer distractions: too much distraction can affect study, especially when preparing for an examination. You want your thought process intact. For some, playing music in the background can be soothing for studying. It doesn't mean starting a singalong session, though. Singing along to the song or fully becoming aware that a song is being played shows one thing, you're distracted, and attention is dissuaded.

Necessary supplies with the right study area: put in materials that will aid your reading. Supplies such as papers, pencils, and pens, rulers, highlighters, a nearby trashcan, can prevent unnecessary movements when these materials are really needed.

Clearing your Calendar for Study

This simply means setting updates or periods of study to prevent clashes with other important events. Dates for important activities like course schedules for topics being introduced and examination commencement are to be noted. Having these in mind will enable you to structure your schedule properly and create time for study.

Choose Appropriate Study Strategy

After setting up good space and time for effective study, the next thing is to get on with it. Yes! But one lingering thought comes to mind after realizing you need to cover lots of information, and that is, where to start from.

Apply these study techniques to help with retaining information:

Identify important areas, ideas, and concepts. To make this easy, glance at the review exercises at the end before you begin the study session. This will expose lots of the main ideas of that assignment, keeping you focused.

Attention on the right topics. You'll be able to learn all there is to know in good time if there is a focus. The type of certification exam offers you the information you need to grasp, and that's some good news.

Chapter 8: How Long Will It Take To Be A Medical Coder?

Actualizing your goal as a medical biller comes with time, and this depends on the chosen career path. The basic requirements for getting started with job applications are your high school diploma or a General Educational Development (GED). If you do not have any experience on the job, make plans to go for an associate degree or certification program to further increase your chances of getting employed.

Programs designed for the medical billing field take about 40-80 hours of course activities, with a time frame of three to six weeks to round up. Some programs are prepared in such a way that you can study the course-work at your convenience, meaning that you can be on the course for a week or up to six months, all depending on you.

The duration of college programs lasts between 2-4 academic semesters, going for 9-21 months. Associate degree programs run for two years, and that of bachelor's degree, four years. Looking at the whole figures, you make up one week to about four years trying to pursue a path to becoming a medical biller. Many individuals interested in the field don't seem to be interested in obtaining a bachelor's degree, so they achieve their aims of becoming a medical biller in two years or maybe less. Running a part-time program is worth considering, but it takes more time to complete an academic program. It can serve as an advantage in a way, though, offering you the opportunity to finish your study at your own pace. With a good educational prerequisite, you have a good chance of securing a good job. Being someone who has a good level of experience in a related field comes with the propensity to get hired without going through additional training programs. There are also accelerated programs with a duration of a few months or even weeks.

After completing all educational requirements, ranging from a program completion or obtaining a certificate, you can then begin your job search.

For medical coders, the period also depends on the route taken to become a professional. If you make a decision to go for certification, diploma, or degree programs, the period it takes to round up such a program will give the time frame. Diploma programs for medical coding can be rounded up in a year. Taking up an associate degree path will see you finish the training and obtain the degree in under two years.

A certification program like the Certified Professional Coder (CPC) requires additional time to meet the required qualifications and take the examination. It is possible to ace the certification examination but lack the required work experience to earn the full status of the CPC. This case will see you getting a CPC Apprentice status until full proof of work experience is provided.

Other considerable factors that can affect the duration of becoming a professional are: how the program is run, online or in person, and the required number of credits. You can pursue an associate or bachelor's degree at a faster rate after running a college program, although this depends on the transfer credits accepted by the school.

Chapter 9: Fundamentals To Assist You With A Medical Billing And Coding Career

You have all opportunities to fully grasp that title of being a medical biller and coder only if you are ready to set your mind and time to train and prepare for it adequately. The strategies below can help find the best school, bag that certification or degree, go for industry certification, search for jobs, and secure a good role in this field.

Make research on the available jobs and check out the specific requirements. This should be done even before going all out to obtain the necessary credentials. Check out the requirements for medical billing and coding roles in your area. Check if they are requesting a particular certification or diploma, or demanding an associate degree.

Decide on a medical billing and coding certificate, diploma, or degree program. Most educational prerequisites fall under these, so take note if preparations for a career are underway. A quick route is going for a diploma program. To give your credentials a boost, consider an associate degree. Put your long-term career goals in mind when making these decisions.

Seek out means of financial assistance. Look out for available scholarships and financial aid programs that you can put in for. These programs help reduce the financial burden, especially if you find it difficult to make school payments. Some schools you're interested in offer scholarships and financial aid.

After graduation, consider going for a certification program. You can, of course, go for medical billing and coding jobs after completing your program, but having the interest to acquire a CPC certification means you'll take the examination. This should be immediately after you graduate or very close to graduation, as the coursework is still in your memory. Also, certification increases your chances of earning decent pay.

Prepare a good resume and go all out to get that job. This is after you've gotten all educational requirements and are fully ready to take up a job role. You can check your school if it offers career services like job search assistants to ease the job search process when applying for local positions.

Go for interviews. You're likely to get called for an interview when potential job employers are satisfied with what is on your resume. Your school career services may have job interviews guides and preparations to improve and hone your interview skills before going for a session. Once you've fully undergone practice sessions, you should then set your mind to go for the real deal.

Accept the job and move up the ladder in your career. On your first job as a professional, it is important you create a good impression at first and live up to the set standards.

Printed in the USA
CPSIA information can be obtained
at www.ICGtesting.com
LVHW010213061023
760342LV00008B/183